My Journey
with MS
A long road

My Journey with MS

The information contained in this book is based on the life experiences and opinions perceived and expressed by the author, Domingos Joaquin Fernandes.

ISBN: 978-1-952070-16-7

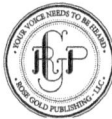

Rose Gold Publishing, LLC
www.RoseGoldPublishingLLC.com

My Journey with MS

"Having a positive state of mind is a great thing;
Putting your mindset at the forefront, the results
may surprise you"

-Domingos Fernandes

My Journey with MS

MY JOURNEY WITH MS

A long road

By

Domingos Joaquin Fernandes

TABLE OF CONTENTS

CHAPTERS

To all the MS patients that have been given an unexpected challenge to adapt to.

Do not be afraid. I promise you; you are not alone. There is always someone there and together, we can give each other hope.

FOREWORD

*W*e have all heard the term 'create your own journey' or 'choose your own path' or 'Just Do It!" All great, inspiring words of advice. But what if your journey suddenly changes, because the universe suddenly decides to CHOOSE a journey for you? Could you handle it? How would you handle it? Would you be ready to give up?

Many of us talk about how we 'overcome' our obstacles in life. Choosing the right 'mindset'. We all have our bad days. What is your 'BAD DAY' compared to others?

My friend of 25 years Domingos Fernandes, or DOM to me, has proven daily that having the right philosophies in your mind, can and DOES make a difference in your achievements in this journey called 'LIFE'. He has been dealing with multiple sclerosis or "MS" for 18 years. Dom has already inspired many around him. His book is not just about educating people about this un-predictable disease. It is not just about the struggles of the disease. Above and beyond those reasons, his book is about living a happy life. A life that can be achieved regardless of what you are dealing with now or where you hope to go with your life.

As a professional talk show host, sports commentator and occasional motivational speaker, I have met thousands of people. While I can take something positive from most of those whom I have met or interviewed, there is only a choice few that I can say have had a tremendous inspiring IMPACT on my life. Dom is one of those people! Dom has reminded me just how powerful our minds can be. That we need to exercise our minds just as much, if not more than our bodies. Aside from his mouth and slight head movement. Dom only has slight movement remaining in his left hand. His choice to continually exercise his mind is PROOF that having the proper philosophies in place, will get you to achieve great things in your journey in life. Dom NEVER complains.

You MUST read this book from start to finish and then keep it out somewhere visible, so that you will always be reminded of your ability to achieve above and beyond in your life's journey.

I am proud to have Domingos Fernandes as my good friend and inspirational projector!

David Burrows
The Show with David Burrows
www.theshowlive.live

ACKNOWLEDGMENT

*T*o all my family, my siblings and children, who have always been there for me, know that I couldn't do this book without you.

To my dear friend David Burrows, who has been in my life since I was 18-years old; your friendship and your love encourage me every day.

To my newest friend, Dolly Cortes, the Owner of Rose Gold Publishing, LLC – thank you for helping me share my story. With you, I know my message will be greatly received.

My Journey with MS

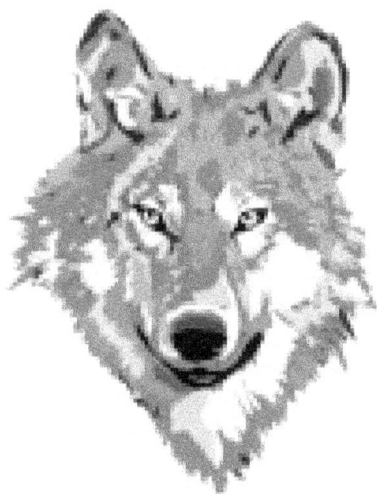

My Journey with MS

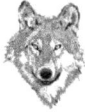

INTRODUCTION

I was born and raised in Sarnia, Canada.

As a healthy young man, I enjoyed sports while in high school, and when I graduated, I worked as a short-order cook. I aspired to be a chef one day. Unfortunately, I couldn't achieve my dream. Actually, I was not able to achieve many of my dreams. My life plan turned out quite different than I had hoped.

At one point, I was also a general laborer and a cab driver but that was also taken away from me.

I loved to sing karaoke, and I recently started singing again. If my health allowed it, I would do it daily. But thanks to technology, I enjoy doing Facebook Live events, and I sing almost daily! I sing with all my heart and I don't care how I sound. It makes me smile because it is fun. I don't care if

I only get one person to hear me. On the contrary, I do it for several reasons; it keeps me active, and I feel that I am inspiring others by not allowing my disease hold be back from doing what I love.

Unless I am in the hospital, I want to keep moving in some way. I want to be heard, seen, and I want to live. You don't realize how lucky you are to be healthy. I miss those days.

My life took a turn when I was diagnosed with Primary Progressive Multiple Sclerosis in January of 2003. I never expected this to happen to me. I certainly did not expect the progression, and at one point, I was terrified and devastated.

This is my story.

My Journey with MS

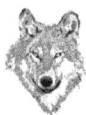

MY STORY

I was 15 years old, and I was riding my bicycle home after visiting a friend when I suddenly began to see double. It seemed that I was getting too close to the road, and I thought I would get hit by a car. I slammed on the brakes so hard that I couldn't help but fall off. As I tried to get up from the ground, I closed each eye individually, and with my left eye, it looked as if I was right next to the road. However, when I closed my right eye, I saw that I was at least 15 feet away from the road. I knew something was wrong. I walked the rest of the way home.

When I arrived at my house, I told my mom what happened, and she immediately called the doctor. My mother made several doctor's appointments, but none of the doctors were able to help. Soon after, I was referred to a neurologist in London. He performed some tests but couldn't find anything wrong. They must have thought it was a fluke, so they suggested waiting a couple of weeks to see if my vision would correct itself, and unfortunately, it did. At that point, no more tests were performed on me.

Doctors today believe that experience was my first Multiple Sclerosis attack.

I was 26 years old. When I heard, "you have MS."

It was hard to hear those words. However, I wasn't just going to accept it. I was only 26! This was not part of my life plan. I wanted to do things. I was not willing to change or to lose everything I wanted, not yet. I wasn't ready. I felt I was at the beginning of my life, not the end, so I honestly struggled with those words. It felt like a death sentence. I didn't know what I did wrong, or why I was being punished this way. I didn't understand why I had to experience this.

Nothing was going as planned. I wanted to have a good life. I wanted to enjoy my family. I wanted to experience life to the fullest as I always had before today, and this, this MS, was not going to take that away!

I decided to ask my neurologist for a second opinion; I needed to make sure. I was hoping they made a mistake; that they were wrong. I was so scared. I didn't want this to be happening to me.

I was referred to the MS clinic in London, and I was nervous about getting the results. I just wondered what my life would be if it were true. How bad will things get? How soon? My mind was filled with questions, and then it happened. Unfortunately, they confirmed it. Honestly, I did not know what to expect, and I was petrified.

In the beginning, I had multiple symptoms, including double vision, loss of balance, and vertigo. I felt out of control. It was so uncomfortable, and it was a difficult experience, it was new to me, and I was a nervous wreck.

For the first few months, I relied heavily on a walker, but it progressed so rapidly that by December of the same year, I was in a wheelchair. I was watching my body lose itself, and there was only so much that I could do. It was beyond my control, and I began to panic. My mind was racing with thoughts. I couldn't believe how fast it was progressing and affecting me.

During this time, I could barely stand and transfer myself out of the wheelchair, but I was becoming weaker. I could also go up and down the stairs on my bum, but that's not what I wanted. I felt helpless. It also felt it was humiliating.

Since so many changes were taking place so fast, I struggled not only with my body but also with severe depression, and although I was able to get my depression under control, it took a number of years and it was probably one of the most difficult times for me and my family.

When a person experiences depression, it's like an additional wrench is thrown at you. Many negative thoughts were going through my head, and I didn't care how those thoughts would hurt me. I was at a point in my life that it was difficult to see the good in any of this. In my opinion, there was absolutely nothing good about my current situation.

This was not how my life was supposed to end. I was angry, hurt, and confused. I didn't know how to deal with this. This was not fair to any of us. I didn't want my family to have to take care of me.

I drowned my sorrows in alcohol, thinking it would help, but it didn't. It made matters worse. I was not very nice or kind to others. So many changes were taking place that I didn't care. My body was losing mobility, and to add salt to my wound, I could not work any longer.

I know it may be difficult to understand, but when a man is not able to work, to provide for his family, it is not only about the paycheck. It is about your sense of failure as a man. I felt I let my family down.

I felt incomplete because I was no longer able to do things as a man should. Being forced to stop working was truly a devastating blow. I felt I lost my freedom. I was so confused and frustrated. I didn't want family or anyone feeling pity for me, and I did not want to ask for help. It hurt. I felt like I was dying slowly inside, and there was nothing I could do. Depending on others to help me made me feel so uncomfortable. I did not want to be a burden. I wanted to live my life without issues. I hated that this happened to me, and I hated to ask for help.

Realizing I did not have many choices, I had to swallow my pride, and I eventually asked for help. I used to be the one to help others, but in an instant, everything changed. I cannot emphasize enough how incredibly uncomfortable I felt. It was great to help others, but it did not feel so good to be the one needing help. I am not sure if you can understand why, but perhaps it was my ego. Life was so complicated then. It was chaotic. I just wanted to live a long, healthy, normal life. This wasn't it.

Also, I was married before to a nice lady, but now we are just best friends. Our marriage was not perfect, but I always wanted her to be happy. I loved her, and I am grateful that she is still in my life.

Today, I have two children of my own, and I raised four stepchildren. I am also a proud step-papa to three beautiful grandchildren. They bring me so much joy, and I love to spend time with them. Until this day, I am happy that my oldest daughter got to know the man I used to be before I became ill. I am so glad today that I am surrounded by them. They visit me regularly and spend time with me.

Unfortunately, MS compromises my immune system daily. It doesn't take much for me to get sick. A simple cough or a sneeze is all it takes. I can feel when something isn't right. When I feel weak or lethargic, I know it's time to get checked.

With MS, I learned to listen to my body. When I feel tired, I take a nap. If I am having a muscle spasm, I try to let it run its course although it is painful. Fighting them only makes them worse. I do realize I am always on the move, though, well as best I can. I don't want to stay still. Perhaps, I want to move because I don't know when it will be the last time. I don't want to miss any part of the day, and I don't want just to be laying in bed waiting for my end to come.

Again, this is not how I was meant to live my life. I had dreams, goals, and expectations. I wanted more than anything to be "normal." I never thought walking would be a luxury I could no longer have. I think about who I am now versus who I used to be. Not being able to feed myself or move around freely; not being able to go for a swim or a drive or to feel free has been extremely difficult.

However, what I eventually realized; God chose me to deal with this. I guess he knew I would figure out a way to not dwell on my existing limitations but on how I can make a difference to others while giving them a message of hope.

I want to share with you three separate conversations that I remember having.

One day, I was at my brother's house for a family gathering; we were in the garage, and my brother said to me, "you're a stronger person than me." I asked, "how so?" he said, "I couldn't deal with what you deal with every day." I told him that I didn't deal with it, but I learned to adapt to the changes instead.

You see, when one is handed a stone, one must decide what to do with it. Do you throw it or save it? Having MS is like saving the stone. I wouldn't throw the stone because it could hurt someone. Instead, I choose to keep it and learn from it. What is my lesson in all of this? I ask myself. After all, my response to the situation doesn't have to be negative. I may not like it but I have accepted it.

On another occasion, during one of my many hospital admissions, a family friend came to visit me. As he was getting ready to leave, he said that he learned something new about me whenever he came to visit.

I asked what he learned that day, and he replied, "that you are very positive, very patient, willing to share your knowledge about your disease." He made me smile. I don't think I realized until then, how I was impacting others while dealing with my condition.

It made me realize that others were paying attention. Therefore, I must be careful in how I deal with my situation. I don't want to show my frustrations or perhaps come across as a negative person. I am a happy person, although I cannot play sports or do the many things that I love. However, I am so grateful to still have experiences with those I love. We have each other, and I couldn't ask for anything better than that.

Another time, I had a friend and her boyfriend over; he asked me a serious question. He asked me if I would rather be in jail with a chance of getting out, or would I rather live the way I am? I told him, "I'd rather be in prison with a chance to get out because, with MS, your body is like being in jail but you will never get out" He was shocked at my answer.

This condition has helped me appreciate all that I have. However, I still miss what I once had. I also regularly think about what could have been. I can't help but wonder. What would my life be like today without MS?

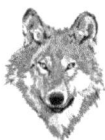

WHAT IS MS?

I want to share what I know about MS with you because I want to make sure that you understand what could potentially happen to your body, mind, and spirit if you have been diagnosed with this disease.

In the beginning, I did not realize what this illness entailed or how, in so many ways, it would affect me. It also affected those around me because without notice, in one way or another, I was surrounded by caretakers.

I am not referring to the hospital staff or the home staff where I reside, but instead of my family and friends. We did not realize how much effort, love, and patience this illness would take from all of us.

I also want to say I am sorry that this has happened to you too.

Multiple Sclerosis, MS, is a disease of the central nervous system. It affects the flow of information between the brain and the body, so not every patient experiences MS the same way since many of the symptoms vary between each patient. Some symptoms are more severe than others, and so is the progression.

A French neurologist named Jean-Martin Charcot discovered Multiple Sclerosis in 1868. He called the discovery "sclerosis en plaques."

There are four types of MS, the most common being Relapsing-Remitting, RRMS.

With this type of MS, the patient may experience eye pain or double vision, numbness, dizziness, and both bowel and bladder problems. When an exacerbation occurs, there is a period of healing.

The second type is called the Second Progressive, SPMS.

Its symptoms include more weakness, stiff leg muscles, issues with bowel and bladder. Patients may experience more challenging times with fatigue, depression, and problems thinking.

The third type of MS is called Primary Progressive, PPMS. This is the type of MS that I was diagnosed with. My symptoms again were double vision, dizziness, vertigo, and overall loss of balance.

I experience severe muscle spasms regularly, muscle tremors, bowel and bladder problems, pins, and needles in my legs along with numbness. The rate of progression varies over time, and it is horrible. Unfortunately, this type is one of the most aggressive forms of MS.

The fourth type of MS is called Progressive Relapsing, PRMS.

Some patients experience eye pain, vision problems, pain in their spine when their neck is bent, bowel and bladder problems.

All forms of MS experience sensitivity to temperature. Some more than others. For example, when temperatures rise above 75 degrees, my body gets so weak that I can't move without assistance. My perfect temperature is about 70 degrees Fahrenheit.

I feel my body freezes up quickly with cold weather, and I also can't move or function. I get muscle spasms, which can be very painful, especially when they create Charlie horses. I am unable to massage my muscles. I don't have mobility in my arms. When I find myself alone and in pain, it is challenging because I can't move. I always need help and must get inside my home to warm up, and I must do it fast because it affects me significantly.

It's sad, but I understand that women are three times more likely to be diagnosed with MS than men. It may have a hormonal tie to the disease.

Primary Progressive Multiple Sclerosis and Progressive Relapsing Multiple Sclerosis are rare forms of the disease, and about 15% of people diagnosed will have PPMS.

On average, it takes about 50% more energy for an MS patient to complete a simple task then it does for an average person. To make matters worse for me, I anxiously await to see what mobility I will lose when I do have an exacerbation. It's my norm. It's interesting. I am so used to this already that I know what to expect. I expect to lose mobility in a new area. As of right now, I can move my head. My mobility to my arms is non-existent. I use my head to push myself in my wheelchair with a joystick. It was a bit challenging to learn to do this, but after so many years, now I consider myself an expert.

MS is known as "Canada's disease" among healthcare professionals because Canada has had and continues to have the highest MS rate in the world.

The United Kingdom has the second-highest rate of MS, with an average of 164 people for every 100,000 diagnosed. Studies show that geography, in general, MS, is more common in areas farthest from the equator.

Globally there are 2.3 million MS patients. Canada's population as of 2017 was 36.71 million people. Of that, 290 people for every 100,000 are diagnosed in Canada. According to the MS Society of Canada, there is an average of 2.9 individuals per 1000 or 1 in 385 Canadians diagnosed daily. The average age of diagnosis is 20 to 49.

There are people older and younger than this being diagnosed as well. When I was diagnosed, the average age of diagnosis was 15 to 26. It seems so much has changed in sixteen years. As of 2012, an estimated 3,800 MS patients live in long-term care facilities in Canada, with another estimated 93,500 MS patients living in private homes.

I'm fortunate to still live independently in my own apartment with assistance from the Ontario March of Dimes. I love living here and the staff of the complex are incredible.

Also, there are disease-modifying drugs for RRMS and SPMS. On February 15, 2018, Health Canada approved a new Disease-Modifying Drug, DMD, for PPMS and RRMS called OCREVUS. This is the first DMD for PPMS. You have to meet specific criteria for this DMD.

So, you know, if you hear an MS patient start to laugh or cry spontaneously at inappropriate times, this is beyond their control. Please don't get upset. On the contrary, I ask you to be patient and understanding. This is called the Pseudobulbar Affect. This is caused when lesions affect the part of the brain that controls emotions. This is also common in other neurological diseases. By the way, the life expectancy of an MS patient is 7 to 10 years less than people without MS.

As of 2017, the life expectancy of a healthy female is 81.2 years, and the life expectancy of a healthy male is 76.2.

As the years go on, I continue to learn and get educated about MS. I think it is necessary. I decided to write this book because I know my experience with MS has been mixed.

There was a time when I was angry, depressed, hating life, and now, it is entirely different. Having MS has made me aware of my body. I still can feel; but I can't move it. I am very attentive, and I try to understand and pay close attention to my triggers.

When I have an exacerbation, I look at it as another obstacle to overcome, and I fight to do so.

Living life with MS has humbled me and given me a new perspective on life. I don't take things for granted anymore. I sincerely appreciate waking up every morning. I get excited to think that I was given another day to share, laugh, and learn.

I encourage you to live life to the fullest because you never know what tomorrow will bring.

While there are many known causes of death in MS patients, such as respiratory failure, cardiovascular disease, infections from pressure sores, suicide is prevalent.

Unfortunately, I shared earlier that I went through a severe depression. However, I was one of the lucky ones. I got better.

Depression does not only affect you, but it also affects those you love, and if you or someone you know is going through a depression, I implore you to seek help.

I also contemplated suicide, but I couldn't do it. I wanted to die because let's be realistic; my future was dark. I didn't see a reason to live. It didn't mean that I didn't have a reason. I had many, but I frankly didn't see it because I was too depressed to notice.

I can only speak for myself, but I am glad I didn't kill myself. If I had, I would not have shared so much with my children. I would not have met my grandchildren. I would not sing and laugh with my buddy, David Burrows! I wouldn't be writing this book or sharing my reality with all of you! I wouldn't be. I would have given up and perhaps have become a whisper in someone's conversation of "poor guy, he couldn't deal with it."

Instead, I am doing the best that I can to cope with this disease. I am pushing myself sometimes to the point of exhaustion. My friends tell me to slow down, but I can't. When I come home from my many hospital visits, I feel I need to jump on my computer and let everyone know; I'm home! Nope, I am not dead yet!

Listen, I ask you to have compassion for others during their time of need. We don't know what a person may be going through. We don't always know their state of mind or what type of day they are having. All we know is what we see on the outside, and even that may be inaccurate.

We need to learn to be kind and loving with one another.

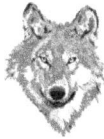

LOSING MOBILITY

I knew it would be difficult for me to cope with my diagnosis. I didn't expect things to happen as quickly as they did. When I was diagnosed with MS, I was not told what to expect. Nothing was explained to me. Can you see how frightening this could be?

Out of nowhere, I remember not being able to move my legs. I had to use my arms to move them physically. I could transfer myself from one place to another, but it wasn't easy, and my knees would buckle.

My struggles were real. My body was losing mobility fast. My oldest child and my stepchildren saw me walk, but my youngest daughter only saw me transfer myself.

I was now experiencing the unknown, and I was scared, so I decided to do some research to understand this condition better. I went online and read every book that I could get my hands on.

I immediately received a lot of support from my family, but this was not easy on them either. This was a significant change. It was not only affecting me physically and emotionally, but it was affecting my family emotionally as well. I remember they helped me find a scooter. They knew it would help me. They try so hard to be by my side, and I am so grateful for them because this is not something, I would wish on anyone. However, having my family by my side makes it easier to deal with. They helped me realize that I was never alone. They are my gift for having this illness. They were there all along, but I never realized how much until I was diagnosed. I learned to appreciate them like never before.

As you know, when I was initially diagnosed, I was upset. I knew my life would never be the same. I soon became depressed. I began to drink. I felt that my life was over, and I contemplated suicide; it was an out. If I couldn't have full mobility of my body, I didn't think I could live like this. I thought it would be an answer, but then the more I thought about it, I realized I didn't want to hurt my family. I knew they loved me. I couldn't be that selfish. I did not want them to go through any pain; they had suffered enough already. But I must admit, I did not want to live this way either. I needed to decide what was more difficult, continuing to live like this, or hurting my family. I would never hurt my family.

In February 2010 I went to Albany, New York, for a controversial treatment called Chronic Cerebral Spinal Venous Insufficiency or CCSVI. An Italian Doctor discovered this by the name of Paulo Zamboni.

Since I wanted my MS to go away, I was hopeful of finding a cure or a treatment. Have you ever seen yourself just desperate about something where you have zero control? That's how I felt. I figured I had nothing to lose other than this disease, so I was willing to try anything.

I lived in the hospital for thirteen months. During my hospital stay, I was doing physiotherapy, occupational therapy, and recreational pool therapy. While doing pool therapy, something incredible happened one day; with help from the therapists, I took my first steps in six and a half years. The therapists started crying, and so did I.

Unfortunately, soon after, I experienced Pulmonary Embolism, (blood clots), and spent a week in telemetry with the most excruciating pain I had ever felt. I was given high doses of blood thinners, and for eight months, I was MS symptom-free. This is not a cure, but those eight months were bliss.

You know, God does work in mysterious ways. I feel that he knew that my first marriage wasn't meant to last however, within two and a half years, of meeting, we were expecting our daughter to be born. We were thrilled. To be blessed with a bundle of joy after doctors told us that I had a 5% chance to father another child because of my MS progression. God gave us a miracle baby that I'm eternally grateful for.

By the way, I have been told repeatedly that I have the patience of Job, a disciple from the bible.

I had marital problems while I was in the hospital for physiotherapy. My condition just caused too much stress for both of us. I didn't expect my marriage to suffer, but it did. We had an amicable breakup and today remain friends. I am grateful she's in my life.

Friends would come and take me to the Grand Bend Motor Plex to watch the drag races. I was picked up one day, and we went to Canatara beach. A friend introduced me to a girl, and she and I hit it off and dated for a while and remain friends to this day.

Unfortunately, being symptom-free was only temporary. Life in the hospital was not fun and games. You're required to be in bed by a specific time and up by another specified time. It was always loud and had very little privacy. If you wanted to leave the floor, you are on or go for a weekend visit; you needed to sign a form called a LOA (Leave of Absence). It records the time that you left and marks the time you come back. I felt a bit belittled by this process. I thought I was being treated like a child. But it was what I needed to do at the time.

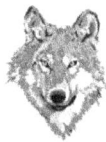

MY ROOMMATES

I became great friends with two of my hospital roommates. As I was about to leave for a LOA, one roommate said to me, "When I feel down, I look over at you, you're always smiling and never grumpy. It makes me feel good and lifts my spirits." I felt humbled when I heard him say that.

Soon after, I had to pick from a list of long-term care facilities and visit them. Hospitals are not meant to be used for the long term. They are only meant to assist you for a short time or immediate need.

I did not have a choice. I had to leave, so I picked a few facilities off the list given to me and went to visit them. I also spoke with a social worker who told me about the Ontario March of Dimes. We put my name on a waiting list for long-term care facilities and the Ontario March of Dimes. The first place I heard from was a long-term care facility, but I wanted to wait to decide until I heard from Ontario March of Dimes because that was my preference. Luckily, they reached out a few days later, and I was able to turn down the long-term care facility. It felt great to have a choice.

I had to go through an interview process with the Ontario March of Dimes and was accepted for their assisted living program to which I was grateful for. I was in my mid-30s at the time. Living here with the Ontario March of Dimes is like living in the hospital but having the privacy of my own home with staff on-site and available 24 hours a day, seven days a week.

Although I left the hospital, I would still visit my roommates when the weather was allowed. My roommates and I made a deal. One week I would buy a basket of apples from the local farmers market, the next week they would buy. I would bring them apples regularly. One day, as the winter weather turned to spring, I went to take them apples, and the nurse in charge stopped me at the desk and asked me who I was there to see. I thought that this was odd as I've never been stopped before. I told her, and at that moment, she informed me, that my roommate passed away. I was deeply saddened by this but knew he was now at peace. He was no longer suffering. He was no longer living, but I knew he was in a better place.

I continued to visit my other roommate, who asked me one day what I liked and collected. I told him wolf memorabilia. I love wolves. He asked for my address, and I obliged. A few weeks passed, and I received a parcel in the mail. It was in a handmade package. I had forgotten about it. On my next visit, I remembered the box and asked what it contained; he told me that it contained CDs with thousands of wolves' pictures. Not long after this visit, he also passed away. To this day, I have not opened the package for sentimental reasons. It makes me sad.

It breaks my heart to see so many people die. It shouldn't be this way. Not like this, not so young.

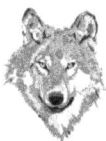

MY TATTOOS

I have tattoos all over my body – eleven of them are "wolves."

A wolf means strength, loyalty, understanding, and intelligence in the native language, and to me, they are majestic. For me, they help me share my story. It is my art and, in a way, my voice.

I need to share my journey and to teach others about MS through my personal experiences.

I am a strong person. I always manage to bounce back, and I don't give up easily. I honestly don't know when to quit although I have my setbacks, I keep coming back, sometimes physically weaker, but always mentally stronger.

I also have vampires and werewolves on my arm sleeve. I enjoy horror films. I enjoy the sting of the tattoo needle. Although it is painful, it is also soothing because it tells me that I can still feel. This feeling gives me a sense of freedom since I don't have it with my body. I find it therapeutic.

I am confined to a wheelchair for the rest of my life. It is my jail, my reality, but it can't stop my thoughts. I am excited to show you a few of my tattoos.

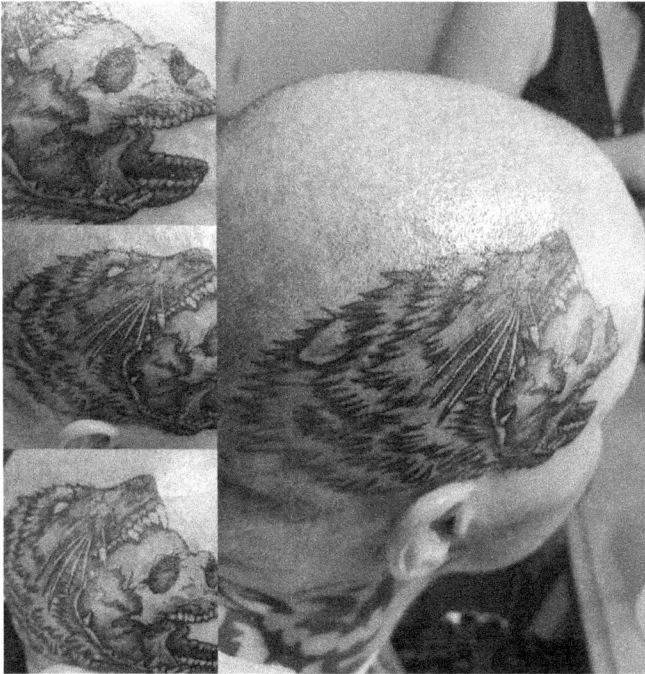

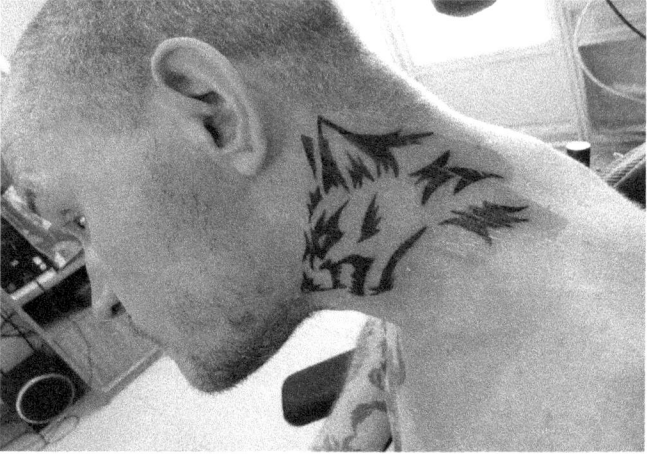

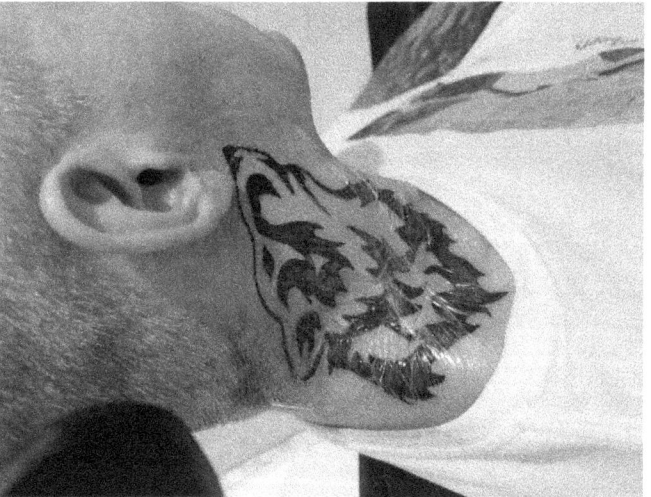

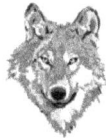

ONTARIO MARCH OF DIMES

*W*hen I first moved into the Ontario March of Dimes assisted living program, I had mixed emotions. I was excited to be moving into my apartment and yet apprehensive, not knowing what to expect. It took some time to adjust. What helped make the transition a bit easier was my next-door neighbor, who happened to be an old high school friend.

I moved in on March 1st, 2012. I made friends rather quickly. The first year living there, I organized a resident's karaoke night. Some sang while the rest watched but everyone had a great time. It was the first time I had ever organized anything, so I enjoyed how well it turned out.

When the weather is beautiful, we all like to congregate outside and talk. Unfortunately, many of the residents, or consumers, as they are referred, come and go. Some have passed away, many of which I was close to. Others go to other programs, so I don't see them again since we don't stay in touch most of the time. I often think of them, I wish them well.

The consumers and the March of Dimes staff may not be blood, but I consider them my extended family. Finding the care and respect that I have found here is second to none. While in the hospital, I was given consideration but no privacy. I feel like this is truly a home for me.

I don't ever think that I would move from here. In 2015 the Ontario March of Dimes wanted to start a local committee here in Sarnia. I stepped up, took on the role of Volunteer Chairman with the option to step down if it became physically challenging. I am happy to say that I am still part of the committee. I feel lucky, I love it, and I don't see myself stepping down anytime soon.

Between 2013 and 2015, I had multiple setbacks. I spent a fair amount of time in the hospital due to the MS exacerbations (attacks). It was challenging, and I must admit that I did go back to drinking during this time. I was not abusing alcohol as it was mainly social, but there were those days that I dealt with frustration and anger. I was tired of the attacks. They were happening too frequently. I was continually getting infections.

I drank until August 5th, 2018, until I was no longer physically able to.

It seems that I was always discharged from the hospital just in time for the Ontario March of Dimes flagship fundraiser "Rock for Dimes." I enjoyed the fundraisers quite a bit. I always wanted to participate in any way that I could.

To this day, the MS attacks have taken a great deal of my mobility, but I fight to keep what movement I have left. I had gone to a tattoo shop one day to make a deposit; a gentleman came into the shop in a wheelchair and asked if I was getting a tattoo. I said I just made a payment. During our conversation, he shared that he was a motivational speaker and as I left the shop, that short conversation kick-started something inside of me that I wanted to do for years, publicly speak about MS. A couple of months later, I started to write a speech. It took me about three months to finish it. I had no idea how to share my speech or who to share it with, but this was my beginning.

I asked a March of Dimes staff member if they had any ideas on how to get started. He suggested I try the MS Society. I thought it was a great idea. I made a phone call, and they gave me two dates to choose from, one in February and the other in June.

I picked February 20th, 2019. I was so excited, but I was so out of my comfort zone.

The day finally arrived, and I was very nervous because not only did I have a live audience, but a very close friend live-streamed my speech for me. I soon realized that the more that I talked, the more relaxed I became.

You see, even with MS, anything is possible when you believe in yourself. There is always hope, and there is still a helping hand.

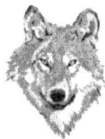

TIPS FOR

ADAPTING TO MS

MS is debilitating and incredibly challenging to deal with at first. However, I found there are ways to adapt to the physical and even emotional pain. I think it is essential to realize that everyone's experience is different, but I hope that my tips will serve someone going through MS.

Below I would like to share some tips that I have used for adapting to MS.

My tips for adapting to MS.

1.   When you first wake up, see how you feel. Your body can predict how your day will go.

2.   Setup an exercise schedule for yourself to help you maintain your mobility but know your limits. Keeping as much mobility that you can as it is to your benefit.

3.   Consider joining support groups through your local MS Society. It can benefit you. Talking to others who are affected by MS, in my opinion, is the best way to learn about this terrible disease.

4.   Find a hobby that will help keep your brain active. I am personally trying to teach myself three languages, Portuguese, Spanish, and French. I host

a support group and a page on Facebook and a talk show called Talking MS. I also enjoy singing, so I do that almost daily.

5. As progression with MS is immanent, you may feel like I did, "My life is over." When you start to feel this way, try this, I was skeptical when I heard this. Sit in a quiet room, close your eyes, breathe deeply through your nose, and slowly exhale through your mouth.

6. Never be afraid to ask for help. Help is always available.

7. Having a support system is essential. Family and friends are a great place to start.

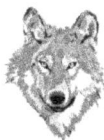

COMFORT ZONE

I started a support group and a support page through Facebook shortly after my first public speaking engagement on February 20, 2019.

I wanted to continue to help those who had questions that needed answering about MS. I wanted this to be a safe haven that nobody is ever turned away from. It was the day I stepped out of my comfort zone.

In April 2019, my good friend, David Burrows, introduced me to live streaming on Facebook. It took me some time to learn how to do it; however, I fell in love with it once I did. I realized it expanded my reach to other countries, so I decided to start my own talk show to reach more people directly.

Through live streaming, I have met some great people internationally, and we have become friends. Live streaming has become one of my favorite hobbies. I've taken this journey and decided to use it to help and motivate others intentionally.

I was once asked, "How is giving back helping you?"

I responded, "It is helping me by giving me a sense of purpose and an overall well sense of being."

Because I decided to share my journey with MS, I have been invited to speak at other locations. I take pride in "not stopping" – the public speaking event will be a joint effort with the MS Society in Canada – they are bringing information for the students – I will speak for roughly 20–30 minutes.

We want the students to be able to ask questions. One of the students used to work here in the March of Dimes program, and she was ecstatic that I was coming to speak – another college also extended this invitation to me.

I love the additional exposure to my message.

This is bigger than me! With MS, if I just laid back and did nothing, it would take over me very fast. Not something that I was willing to do.

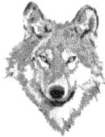

WHERE I AM TODAY

*W*aking up every day for me is a blessing. I am so happy to be alive. Many people don't realize what they have until they lose it. They often take things for granted, and when they no longer have it, they struggle. I used to be that person. I struggled, but now I am so appreciative and grateful for everything and everyone in my life.

I look at life from a different lens. I look forward to doing my daily shows, to talking to other people from different parts of the world, and I can't get enough of my family.

I try to help others daily. I will share my message; in fact, the other day, I was singing! I was singing. I felt fantastic; I felt alive! I felt the music inside, and although I could not lift myself from this chair and dance, the music brought me joy. And I loved sharing my song with those that listened to me that day.

I am a lucky guy. I didn't know it at first, but I am.

People have been so good and kind to me, not because they feel sorry for me but because they love me, and I know it. I feel it.

Do I wish to be able to walk and to dance and to run or to drive? Of course! I miss it. But not being able to do those things has allowed me to do other things, making me happier.

I love the hugs I get from my friends and family. I love that they have always supported me and believed in me. I love that they didn't give up on me even when I was not very nice to them!

I believe I am a better man now then I was before. I have learned to appreciate those that surround me and all that I have. Now, all I want to do is help people every day. This fills me. This makes me happy because I know I am making a difference in their lives. I don't know what kind of day a person may be having, but I know that it may impact and help them by just sharing a positive message. The ability to give back is freeing.

People tell me I inspire them. I was surprised when I first heard it, but then I heard it again, and I started to believe it.

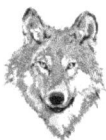

THE LADYBUG

*A*pproximately four years ago, my friend Sandra gave me a small ladybug as a gift. It's not alive, but the meaning behind it is.

A ladybug never gives up and is strong. It also focuses on good fortune, love, and innocence. To me, this ladybug reminds me every day how I must not give in to the discomforts, the pain, including the inconveniences that this illness continually reminds me of.

I am confident when Sandra gave me this token; she could not imagine how dear it would be to me.

Daily, as I sit in front of my computer desk, I look at it. I am grateful to have it.

This ladybug symbolizes strength, and I want to be like her. I don't want to be considered a weak man because I can't walk or am limited.

I want to demonstrate to the world that although I have MS, it doesn't have me. I will continue to stand my ground and share my messages daily to those willing to listen.

Writing this book has been such an incredible journey. It is my way to ensure that my voice is heard now and continues to be heard for generations to come.

Giving up is not an option for me, and I am not going to lie; there have been many moments when I am taken to the hospital, and I can't help but wonder if I will come back home. I have been afraid of the idea not because I am not ready, but because it's too soon!

I am not done creating a better world for myself and those that I love. I am also not done sharing my experiences to help others.

Like the ladybug, I must continue to be strong and persevere, so those who follow me could have a better and clearer path one day.

I never wanted to be a burden to my family, and I am sorry if I have. Just know that within me is a man that stands tall and is proud to live.

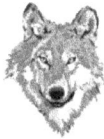

MY MESSAGE TO YOU

*L*iving with MS has been the most challenging thing I have had to endure in my life. Based on what I have shared with you so far, it has been devastating in so many ways, and yet, it has been an absolute blessing.

I wish with all my heart that I was not diagnosed with MS. I wish I could get up and walk around my apartment. I would love to go to the store or go swimming or go for a drive, but my life was not meant to be lived this way.

My life was meant to have challenges, and I don't know why this had to happen to me, but I am grateful that it did, and I will explain to you why.

Again, living my life with MS has been difficult, but you know what it showed me and gave me?

MS gave me a family that I love and am proud of. MS gave me genuine friends that are there for me when I need them. I am not surrounded by people that want to use me or take advantage of me.

MS made me responsible. It made me accountable for sharing my story. It made me responsible for letting others know that life was not meant to be easy, but it was meant to be lived. I could have taken the easy way out. I could have killed myself just like many other MS patients that couldn't handle it did. I chose not to because although I am bound to a wheelchair, it is my responsibility to inform others of what it is like. I am responsible for letting you know that if you are having a bad day or a bad week or month, I have lost control of my body, but I am still smiling.

Stop giving up and dwelling on your past. Choose today to make a difference not only for yourself but for those you love. Or make a difference because you can.

To live is not to have a perfect life. To live life to its fullest is knowing that you don't know what tomorrow has in store for you. I may not wake up tomorrow. I realized that a while ago. Every morning when I open my eyes, I tell myself it's going to be a wonderful day. I am grateful to have one more day, and as I write this book, I have been in the hospital many times, and I don't know if my next visit to the hospital will be the last one.

I have attacks regularly. I have infections regularly, as well. I can't eat on my own, get dressed or even

bathe on my own, but how cool is it that I have people that want me to live and to be there in their lives and therefore, they make it possible for me to be here with you today and to share my experiences.
Living is what life is all about. LIVE today before it is too late.

Everything that could have gone wrong in my life has, and yet I am still smiling.

I lost my dream of being a cook. I can no longer drive. I can't swim. I can't get up from my bed and serve myself a cup of coffee. I got divorced. I drank. I became depressed, and oh yes, I have MS. I also have my amazing kids and beautiful grandchildren.

I still have a heart, a beating heart. I have emotions, and I love my life. I love what I do every day in every way.

I hope that my story brings you hope, as that is my dream.

I don't want to be remembered as an MS patient that lived in a wheelchair. Instead, I want to be remembered as Domingos Fernandes, a man that loved life until the very end and made sure everyone knew it.

As you can see, my journey with MS has not been an easy one, but an intentional one. I am not a victim, but for now, a survivor.

Being diagnosed with MS at such an early age was not what I had ever hoped for my life, but it was God's will.

I hope that sharing my story with you will allow you the peace that perhaps you are seeking. I also hope that your journey is not as physically painful as mine has been if you are a patient.

If you are not a patient, but you know someone, I ask you to please gift a copy of this book to that person. I promise you; you may change that person's life for the better.

Again, MS chose me, I would never have chosen to live this way, but I am grateful that my experiences can help someone else.

Most importantly, I am grateful for those that have stood by my side. Without you, I wouldn't be where I am today!

I love you all,

Domingos Joaquin Fernandes

"The key to living a peaceful, happy life,
is positivity"

-Domingos Fernandes

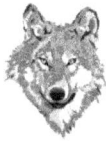

MEMORIES

In the following pages, I will share some of my favorite memories that keep me going every day.

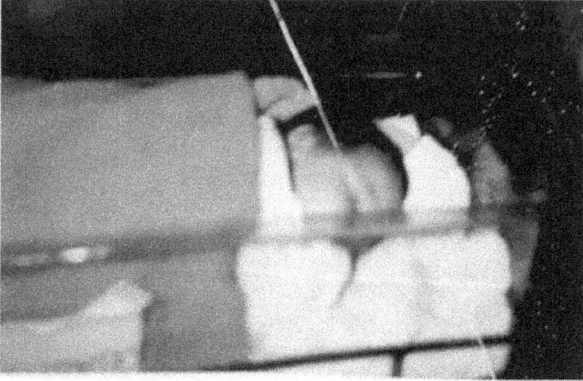

This was me as a child. I love this picture
because I look so innocent and in peace.

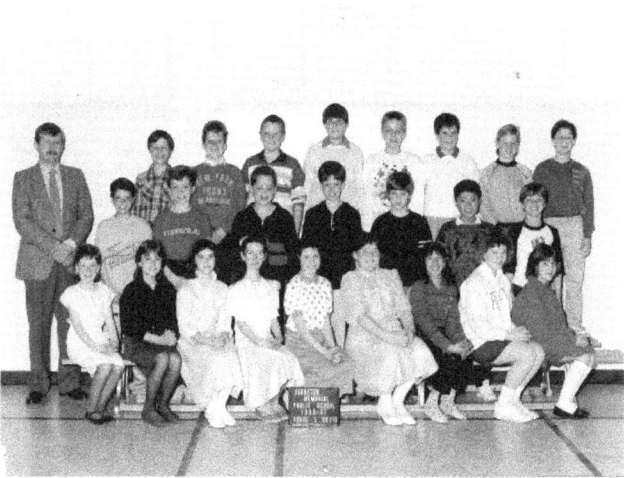

This is my fifth-grade class picture.
I was young and obviously healthy.

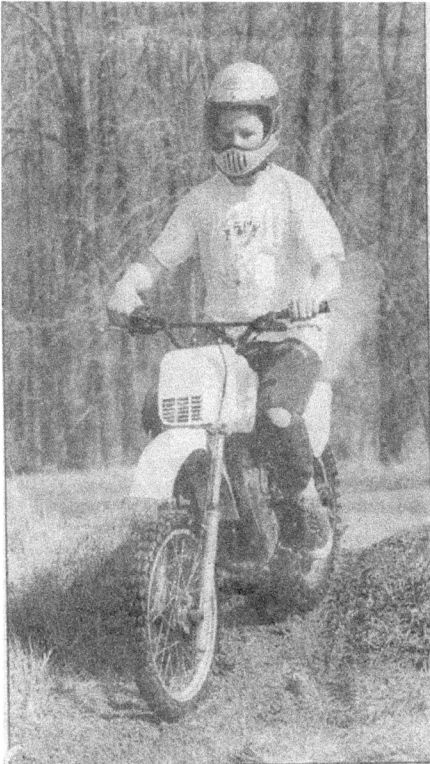

Takes to the hills

Dominic Fernandes, 18, takes to the hills during March Break from Alexander Mackenzie School. The Grade 11 student was spotted on his friend's Yamaha 80 motorcross bike circling the rugged open field at Confederation and Finch Drive.

I used to take risks and was adventurous. I had a zest for life, and I lived every day in the best way.

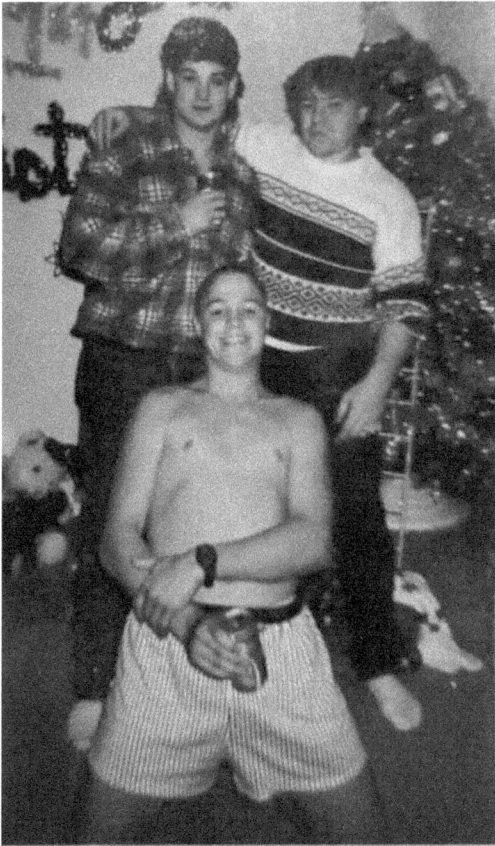

I am always happy! I love this picture,
it represents my energy, my nature, my truth.

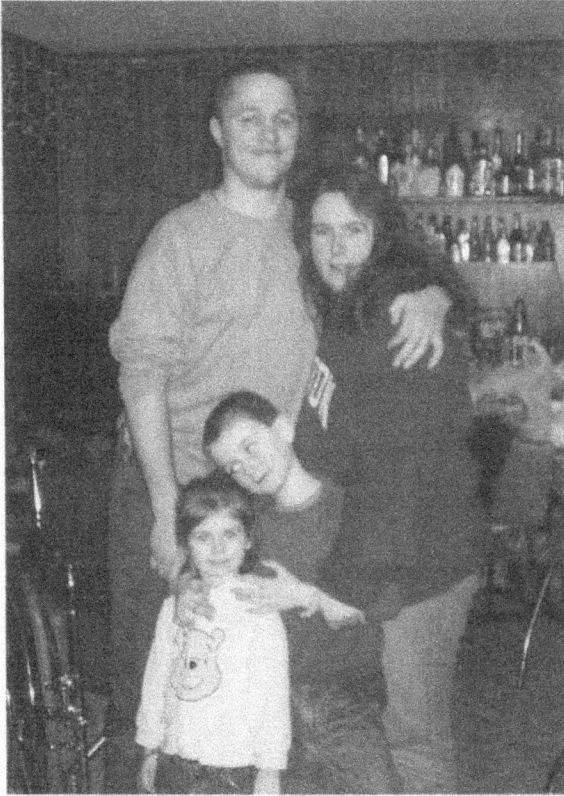

My ex-common law wife and my two stepchildren. I love them all. This is one moment that I was able to stand on my own. As you can see, the wheelchair is immediately behind me. My MS did not have as much control of me as it does now.

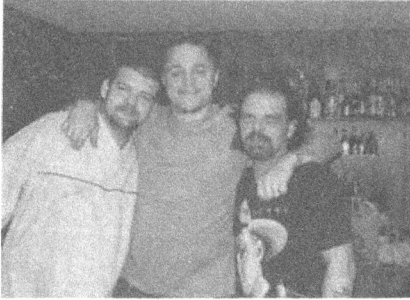

I am still taller than them!

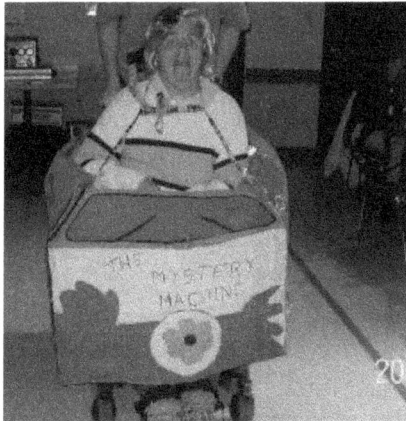

I can't help but smile when I see this picture! I love life. I can't help but enjoy and be grateful for all that I have.

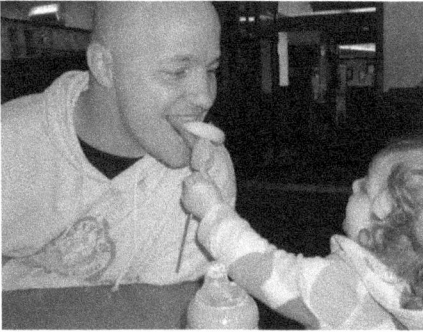

She was feeding me lemons
and I loved every minute of it.

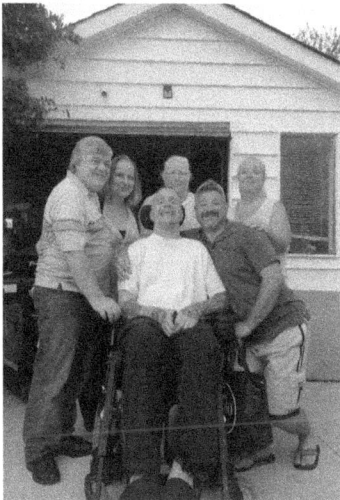

I am surrounded by those I love.

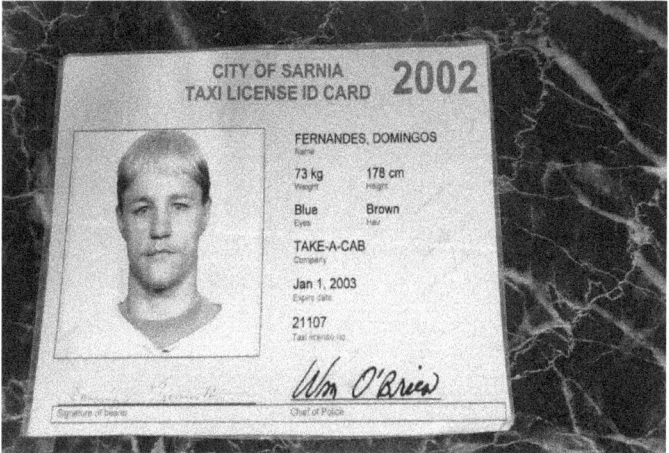

My Taxi ID Card from 2002.
I loved being a cab driver.
I really enjoyed the freedom driving gave me.
It was more than a job, it

Guided
Christmas Card Making

Join the MS Society
to make your own Christmas cards.

Feel like you're not physically able to make a Christmas card?
Don't worry you can bring someone to assist you
and there will be volunteers on hand to assist.

Come out for some laughs and good times.

You'll have a keepsake to boot.

Free to MS Society Community

Sarnia
November 12, 2019
9:30 - 11:00 a.m.
MS Society Sarnia Office
420 East Street Sarnia, ON

To RSVP Call 1-888-510-7777
or email wendi.anderson@mssociety.ca

In 2019, I decided to do something fun, and I got involved in making my own Christmas cards and sold them. I really enjoyed it.

I never want to sit around without doing anything; I need to keep my mind and heart moving. I lost my mobility but not my life. I know that the cards I created brought others joy. Although I am confined to my wheelchair, I feel proud that I can make a difference in other people's lives,

★ ★ ★

My Journey with MS

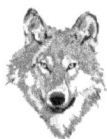

Q & A

I wanted to share some of the many questions that my publisher asked of me during this journey. I think it is nice to share what was happening behind the scenes.

What is your ultimate goal with sharing your story?

To inspire others to share their story – talk to other MS patients and let them know they are not alone.

If there was a cure for MS, what would be the first thing you would do as you walk away from that wheelchair?

Find the nearest swimming pool and dive in! I used to enjoy swimming with all my friends. I can't do physical therapy in water due to the catheter and the water having chlorine – it can cause severe issues.

What do you miss the most since being diagnosed?

I miss driving the most. I would jump in the car and drive around aimlessly. That's why I became a cab driver.

When you realized that you were no longer able to drive, what did that do to you?

It was devastating yet expected. I hated that something I loved was taken away so quickly. I did not want to accept it at first, but that was my new reality.

Was driving peaceful to you?

Yes, and it gave me ample opportunity to get out. It was a love for my freedom. I don't have the freedom that I used to. It is out of my control. Losing my ability to drive was a hard pill to swallow; it was tough to accept it.

If you could change something today, what would that be?

Making mistakes when I was able-bodied – I knew they were wrong, but I did them anyway. I reached out to some people that I hurt way back when and offered them an apology. Some people were surprised that I would apologize.

How would you feel of those that wouldn't accept your apology?

Not everyone accepted my apology – more like forget about it – it happened so many years ago. I guess they thought, poor guy, let it go.

Do you think people feel sorry for you?

My biggest pet peeve – people assume I was in an accident. Some people would say "sorry" that you have MS.

I don't want a pity party. I accept people saying they are sorry, but it is not necessary.

Why does it bother you that they think it is an accident?

The fact that they automatically jump to the accident assumption. Then the conversation ends.

It becomes an awkward moment.

Why do you think that is?

I have an no idea.

What was a dream that you didn't accomplish?

I wanted to get my black belt in Tae Kwon Do, but that was when I finished HS.

Once the MS kicked in, I was not able to become a chef. I used to be a short-order cook. I really enjoyed cooking.

As a short-order cook, I shared my knowledge with the staff. Everyone knew the staff was cooking my meals my way because they could smell it.

You wanted to share your favorite dish with us…do you have the recipe?

My favorite dish is Portuguese shrimp because of the spice.

Here is the recipe:

Ingredients

2 lbs large raw shrimp, with the shell & deveined

1 small onion, finely chopped

3 garlic cloves, minced

5 sprigs parsley, finely chopped

1 teaspoon paprika1 teaspoon salt

1 chicken bouillon cube

1 $\frac{1}{2}$ teaspoons hot pepper sauce (or to taste)

1 $\frac{1}{2}$ teaspoons tomato paste

1 (10 ounce) bottle beer

oil (enough to cover the base of the pan)

In a large frying pan with oil, sauté the onions and garlic for several minutes. Add all the spices, parsley, chicken bouillon, tomato paste, pepper sauce, and half of the beer and let the sauce simmer for approximately 5 minutes.

Once simmered, add the shrimp and remaining beer. Taste the sauce and adjust the seasonings to suite your taste. Once the sauce has been absorbed by the shrimp and the shrimp have turned pink, remove from the pan and serve.

Domingos, are you really happy?

I am. Life hasn't been easy, but I know my family loves me, and I have many friends. That makes me extremely happy.

Are you afraid to die?

No. I am not afraid to die, but I am fearful of leaving my family behind. I also don't want to die. I am young. I want to live; I feel I can still do so much more.

What message do you want to give to your family?

I want my family to know that I love them very much. Without them, I would not have been able to cope with MS the way I have. I am grateful for their patience and their love.

I am grateful they allowed me just to be me. I know I can be silly sometimes, and perhaps an inconvenience, but I believe they respect me and genuinely care about me.

I also want to let them know that they make me happy. I often smile because of the memories we have shared, and because they don't leave my side. I am genuinely grateful.

Please know that I will be donating a percentage of the proceeds from the book sales to the MS Society of Canada. I want to assist with their programs and services but most importantly in funding MS research.

I want to be able to support them any way that I can. Their contributions to my life and many other patients are invaluable, and I want them to know how much I appreciate them.